Breathing Easy

Navigating Life with Asthma

Rossana Lewis

TABLE OF CONTENT

Chapter 1: Understanding Asthma

1.1 What is Asthma?

Asthma, also called bronchial asthma, is a disease that affects your lungs. It's a chronic (ongoing) condition, meaning it doesn't go away and needs ongoing medical management.

Asthma affects more than 25 million people in the U.S. currently. This total includes more than 5 million children. Asthma can be life-threatening if you don't get treatment.

What is an Asthma Attack?

When you breathe normally, muscles around your airways are relaxed, letting air move easily and quietly. During an asthma attack, three things can happen:

- Bronchospasm: The muscles around the airways constrict (tighten). When they tighten, it makes your airways narrow. Air cannot flow freely through constricted airways.

- Inflammation: The lining of your airways becomes swollen. Swollen airways don't let as much air in or out of your lungs.

- Mucus production: During the attack, your body creates more mucus. This thick mucus clogs airways.

When your airways get tighter, you make a sound called wheezing when you breathe, a noise your airways make when you breathe out. You might also hear an asthma attack called an exacerbation or a flare-up. It's the term for when your asthma isn't controlled.

1.2 Types and Triggers of Asthma

If you have asthma, knowing which type you have can help you manage it better.

Allergic Asthma: Allergic asthma, sometimes called atopic asthma, is asthma triggered by allergens like pollen, pets, and dust mites. About 80% of people with asthma have allergies.

Seasonal Asthma: Some people have asthma that only flares up at certain times of the year, such as during hay fever season, or when it's cold. While asthma is usually a long-term condition, it's possible to be symptom-free when your triggers aren't around. It's still important to keep following your asthma action plan and to take your preventer inhaler as prescribed. If you've been diagnosed with seasonal asthma, or think you have it, speak to your GP or asthma nurse about the best ways to manage it.

Occupational Asthma: Occupational asthma is asthma caused directly by the work you do. You might have occupational asthma if:

- your asthma symptoms started as an adult and
- your asthma symptoms improve on the days you're not at work.

Occupational asthma can be caused by many things. For example, if you work in a bakery, flour dust could trigger symptoms, or if you work in healthcare, latex might be a trigger.

Non-allergic Asthma: Non-allergic asthma, also known as non-atopic asthma, is asthma that isn't related to an allergy trigger like pollen or dust. It's less common than allergic asthma. Non-allergic asthma often develops later in life. If your asthma does not seem to be triggered by things like pollen, dust mites or pets, you might have non-allergic asthma.

Exercise-induced Asthma: About 90% of people with asthma have tightening of the airways caused by exercise. However, this can also occur in people without asthma. If you don't have a diagnosis of asthma, but you're getting symptoms like a tight chest, breathlessness, coughing, or fatigue during or after exercising, see your GP.

Childhood Asthma: Some children diagnosed with asthma find it improves or disappears completely as they get older. This is known as childhood asthma. However, it can sometimes return later in life.

Triggers of Asthma
Allergens: Pollen, mold, dust mites, pet dander, and cockroach droppings are common allergens that can trigger asthma symptoms.

Respiratory Infections: Viral infections like the common cold, flu, or respiratory syncytial virus (RSV) can exacerbate asthma symptoms.

Environmental Factors: Exposure to irritants such as smoke, strong odors, air pollution, or sudden weather changes can trigger asthma attacks.

Exercise: Physical activity, particularly in cold or dry air, can induce exercise-induced bronchoconstriction (EIB), leading to asthma symptoms during or after exercise.

Stress and Emotions: Emotional stress or extreme emotions can sometimes trigger asthma symptoms or worsen existing ones.

Medications: Some medications, such as aspirin or nonsteroidal anti-inflammatory drugs (NSAIDs), and beta-blockers, can trigger asthma symptoms in susceptible individuals.

Occupational Exposures: Working in environments with dust, chemicals, gases, or fumes can trigger occupational asthma.

1.3 How Asthma Affects the Respiratory System

The respiratory system has numerous components, and asthma may affect all of them in some way. Here's what this system involves and how asthma might have an impact.

Mouth: With breathing challenges, there's a tendency to breathe through the mouth, which can dry out the mucus membranes there; that may increase risk of cavities as well as an oral yeast infection, called thrush.

Nose: Many people with asthma also have issues with their nose and sinuses due to inflammation and swelling within the sinus cavity. This can lead to chronic congestion that makes breathing even more difficult.

Larynx: Also called the voicebox, this can become hypersensitive when you have asthma, leading to increased cough or vocal cord dysfunction, which can make it hard to breathe.

Trachea: Also called the windpipe, this is a smooth muscle that brings oxygen to your lungs. Similar to other airways, it can become inflamed and constricted due to asthma. That might reduce how much oxygen you can take into the body, reducing the amount that reaches the lungs.

Airways: These are composed of both the small airways (bronchioles) and large airways (bronchi). During an asthma attack, the muscles lining both types of airways can contract, causing them to narrow and become inflamed. If there's also an increase in mucus, which is common with asthma, the bronchioles may get blocked.

Lungs: With asthma there is always at least some swelling within the lungs due to inflammation. That can worsen breathing and make it difficult to take deep breaths. If you're coughing or wheezing, that can exacerbate inflammation and mucus production.

Chapter 2: Signs, Symptoms and Diagnosis

2.1 Recognizing Asthma Symptoms

Asthma symptoms can differ for each person, but here are some of the most common:

Wheezing: You may notice a whistling sound when you breathe. Sometimes this happens only when you exercise or have a cold.

Frequent cough: This may be more common at night. You may or may not cough up mucus.

Shortness of breath: This is the feeling that you can't get enough air into your lungs. It may occur only once in a while, or often.

Chest tightness: Your chest may feel tight, especially during cold weather or exercise. This can also be the first sign of a flare-up.

2.2 Diagnostic Tests and Procedures

Your doctor will use tests to diagnose asthma. Some measure how well your lungs work. Others can tell if you're allergic to mold, pollen, or other things.

All of these asthma tests help your doctor decide if you have asthma and other conditions that often come with it, like allergies, GERD, and sinusitis.

Physical Exam

Your doctor will start with a physical exam. They will:

- Look at your nose, throat, and upper airways
- Use a stethoscope to listen for a whistling sound when you breathe
- Check your skin for allergy symptoms like eczema or hives

They'll also ask you about signs of asthma such as:
- Wheezing
- Coughing
- Breathing problems
- Chest tightness

Medical History

Next, your doctor will ask about your symptoms and overall health to figure out if asthma or something else is causing your problem. Some questions might include:

- What are your symptoms?
- When do you have them?
- What seems to trigger them? What about cold air, exercise, or allergies?
- Do you have hay fever or allergies?
- Does a family member have hay fever, asthma, or allergies?
- What other health problems do you have?
- What medications do you take?
- Do you often come into contact with tobacco smoke, pets, dust, or chemicals in the air?
- What do you do for a living?

Lung Function Tests

Lung function tests are a way to check how well your lungs are working. Doctors use them to diagnose asthma and to monitor its progression. Monitoring asthma with lung function tests is helpful, because you may not always be able to tell just from your symptoms whether your asthma is under control.

In most cases, you have lung function tests in an exam room that contains special devices to measure lung function. A specially trained respiratory therapist or technician is likely to do the tests.

Ask your doctor if you should do anything to prepare for your lung function tests. For instance, you might need to adjust your medication. You may also need to avoid heavy meals, smoking, and any irritants or other substances that might trigger an asthma attack.

Types of Lung Function Tests

These lung function tests are commonly used to diagnose and monitor asthma:

Spirometry is the most common. It's a simple, quick, and painless way to check your lungs and airways. You take a deep breath and exhale into a hose attached to a device called a spirometer. It records how much air you blow out (called forced vital capacity or FVC) and how quickly you do it (called forced expiratory volume or FEV). Your score is lower if your airways are swollen or constricted because of asthma or other lung diseases. Your doctor may want you to have several spirometry lung function tests to monitor your asthma over time. You might have spirometry before and after you take medication to see if the medication helps. Your doctor may also want readings taken during exercise to see how your airways react to exercise.

Challenge tests are lung function tests used to help confirm a diagnosis of asthma. You inhale a small amount of a substance known to trigger symptoms in people with asthma, such as histamine or methacholine. After inhaling the substance, someone tests your lung function. Because challenge tests can trigger an asthma attack, you should have them done only by someone with experience.

Peak flow meter tests measure how well your lungs push out air. Although they are less accurate than spirometry, these lung function tests can be a good way to regularly test your lung function at home -- even before you feel any symptoms. A peak flow meter can help you know what makes your asthma worse, whether treatment is working, and when you need to seek emergency care. The peak flow meter is a handheld plastic tube with a mouthpiece on one end, which you breathe into. Your doctor might ask you to use the peak flow meter each day and write down the readings. After a couple of weeks, you report the results to your doctor.

Exhaled nitric oxide test. You'll breathe into a tube connected to a machine that measures the amount of nitric oxide in your breath. Your body makes this gas normally, but levels could be high if your airways are inflamed.

Other Tests You May Need if You Have Asthma
Even if your lung function tests are normal, your doctor may order other tests to see what could be causing your asthma symptoms.

Gas and diffusion tests can measure how well your blood absorbs oxygen and other gases from the air you breathe. You breathe in a small amount of a gas, hold your breath, then blow out. The gas you exhale is analyzed to see how much your blood has absorbed.

X-rays may tell if there are any other problems with your lungs, or if asthma is causing your symptoms. High-energy radiation creates a picture of your lungs. You may be asked to briefly hold your breath while you stand in front of the X-ray machine.

2.3 Differentiating Asthma from Other Respiratory Conditions

Asthma vs. Chronic Obstructive Pulmonary Disease (COPD):

Similarities: Both asthma and COPD can cause breathing difficulties, coughing, wheezing, and chest tightness.

Differences: Asthma often starts in childhood or early adulthood and is characterized by reversible airway obstruction, whereas COPD usually develops later in life due to long-term exposure to irritants like cigarette smoke, with irreversible airflow limitation.

Asthma vs. Allergic Rhinitis (Hay Fever):

Similarities: Both conditions may involve nasal congestion, sneezing, and itchy, watery eyes.

Differences: Asthma primarily affects the lower airways, causing wheezing and shortness of breath, while allergic rhinitis affects the upper airways, causing symptoms primarily in the nose and eyes.

Asthma vs. Bronchitis:
Similarities: Both conditions can cause coughing and chest discomfort.

Differences: Asthma is a chronic condition characterized by reversible airflow obstruction, while bronchitis is often acute and involves inflammation of the bronchial tubes due to viral or bacterial infections.

Asthma vs. Pneumonia:
Similarities: Both conditions may involve coughing and difficulty breathing.

Differences: Asthma is a chronic condition characterized by inflammation and narrowing of the airways, while pneumonia is an acute infection in the lungs often accompanied by fever, chills, and productive cough with mucus.

Asthma vs. Pulmonary Embolism:
Similarities: Both conditions can cause shortness of breath.

Differences: Asthma involves airway inflammation and narrowing, while a pulmonary embolism is caused by a blood clot blocking a pulmonary artery, leading to sudden and severe shortness of breath, chest pain, and coughing up blood.

Asthma vs. Upper Respiratory Infections (URIs):

Similarities: Both asthma and URIs can cause coughing and breathing difficulties.

Differences: Asthma is a chronic condition with recurrent symptoms, while URIs are temporary infections of the upper respiratory tract caused by viruses.

Chapter 3: Managing Asthma Attacks

3.1 Immediate Action Plan During an Attack

Stay Calm: Remain as calm as possible. Panic can worsen breathing difficulties. Sit in an upright position to help ease breathing.

Use Inhaler Promptly:

- Take your quick-relief medication (short-acting bronchodilator) immediately. Follow the dosage prescribed in your asthma action plan.
- If using a Metered-Dose Inhaler (MDI), shake it, exhale gently, and then inhale the medication slowly and deeply. Hold your breath for about 10 seconds before exhaling.

- For a Dry Powder Inhaler (DPI), follow the instructions for loading the dose and inhale the medication swiftly and deeply.

Use a Spacer if Available:

- If you have a spacer device with your inhaler, use it. Spacers help ensure the medication reaches your lungs effectively, especially for those who find it challenging to coordinate inhalation with the spray.

Monitor Your Breathing:

- Assess your breathing. If symptoms persist or worsen after the first dose, do not hesitate to take additional puffs as directed in your asthma action plan.

Stay Prepared:

- Ensure your inhaler and action plan are easily accessible and known to those around you. Carry your action plan with emergency contacts and instructions for quick reference.

Do Not Delay Seeking Help:

- If symptoms do not improve after taking the inhaler or if there's a rapid deterioration in breathing, seek immediate medical assistance.
- Call emergency services or proceed to the nearest emergency room if experiencing severe breathing difficulties or if you are unable to speak due to breathlessness.

Assist Others if Necessary:

- If you witness someone having an asthma attack and they are unable to manage it themselves, assist them by locating their inhaler and following their action plan. Call for emergency assistance if the situation worsens.

Maintain Calm Breathing Techniques:

- Continue to take slow, deep breaths while awaiting medical help. Keeping calm and controlling breathing as much as possible is beneficial.

Follow-Up With Healthcare Provider:

- After the attack has been managed or once you receive medical care, follow up with your healthcare provider for a review and potential adjustments to your asthma action plan.

3.2 Using Inhalers and Medications Effectively

Effectively managing asthma involves understanding and using inhalers and medications correctly. Inhalers come in various types, such as Metered-Dose Inhalers (MDIs) and Dry Powder Inhalers (DPIs). To use MDIs effectively, one should shake the inhaler, breathe out gently, and then inhale slowly while pressing the inhaler. Holding the breath for 10 seconds before exhaling helps the medication reach the lungs. DPIs require a quick, deep inhalation to ensure the powder reaches the lungs.

Using spacer devices with MDIs can improve medication delivery, particularly for individuals who struggle with coordination. Adherence to the prescribed schedule for long-term controllers, like inhaled corticosteroids, is vital for managing chronic inflammation. Quick-relief medications, or short-acting bronchodilators, offer immediate relief during acute symptoms but should not substitute long-term controllers.

Regular check-ups with healthcare providers help assess asthma control, adjust medications, and address concerns. Developing an emergency action plan is crucial, outlining when and how to use medications during exacerbations. Additionally, maintaining inhalers by keeping them clean, replacing them as recommended, and storing them correctly ensures their effectiveness.

Educating family members, friends, or caregivers about asthma emergencies is also essential. By following these practices and collaborating closely with healthcare providers, individuals with asthma can effectively manage their condition, ensuring proper technique, adherence, and overall optimal asthma control.

3.3 Emergency Preparedness and When to Seek Medical Help

Managing asthma involves being prepared for emergencies and knowing when to seek immediate medical assistance. Here's a comprehensive guide to emergency preparedness for individuals with asthma:

Creating an Asthma Action Plan: An asthma action plan, developed in collaboration with a healthcare provider, serves as a personalized guide. It outlines daily management strategies and specific steps to take during worsening symptoms or emergencies. This plan should be easily accessible and shared with family, caregivers, and close contacts.

Recognizing Signs of an Asthma Emergency: Understanding the signs indicating an emergency is vital. Severe shortness of breath, inability to speak due to breathlessness, chest pain or tightness, bluish lips or fingernails, and a rapid pulse are indicators of a potential emergency. Recognizing these signs is crucial for prompt action.

Using Quick-Relief Medications: During an asthma attack, the use of quick-relief medications (short-acting bronchodilators) as prescribed in the action plan is essential.

Administering these medications promptly can help alleviate symptoms and prevent the situation from worsening.

Immediate Steps During an Asthma Attack: Remaining calm and sitting upright while taking slow, deep breaths is recommended. It's crucial to use the inhaler as directed and ensure it is readily accessible. If available, using a spacer with the inhaler can optimize the delivery of medication to the airways.

When to Seek Emergency Medical Help: If symptoms persist or worsen after using the inhaler, or if there's a rapid deterioration in breathing, seeking emergency medical assistance is imperative. Contacting emergency services or visiting the nearest emergency room is crucial, especially in cases of severe breathing difficulties or when an individual is unable to speak due to breathlessness.

Preparedness at Home: Having emergency contact numbers readily available, including those of your doctor, local emergency services, and the nearest hospital, is essential. Storing prescribed medications, including inhalers, in an easily accessible place ensures quick access during emergencies.

Communicating with Caregivers and Family: Informing family members, caregivers, or close friends about your asthma action plan and the necessary steps to take during an emergency is vital. Educating them on recognizing emergency signs and the proper use of medications can be lifesaving.

Follow-Up Care: After experiencing an asthma emergency, following up with a healthcare provider is crucial. Reviewing the incident, making necessary adjustments to the action plan, and implementing measures to prevent future emergencies are essential steps for ongoing asthma management.

Chapter 4: Lifestyle Modifications for Asthma Management

4.1 Identifying and Avoiding Triggers

Like we explained in chapter 1, asthma triggers are materials, conditions, or activities that either worsen asthma symptoms or cause an asthma flare-up. Asthma triggers are common, which is precisely what makes them so troublesome.

In some cases, avoiding all of your asthma triggers can be difficult. However, with a little planning, you can learn to prevent exposure to your triggers and reduce your risk for an asthma flare-up or attack.

Triggers in the Air

Exposure to pollen, air pollution, cigarette smoke, and fumes from burning vegetation can make your asthma flare up. Pollen is most troublesome during spring and fall, although flowers, weeds, and grasses bloom throughout the year. Avoid being outside during peak pollen times of day.

Use air conditioning if you have it. Air conditioning reduces indoor air pollutants, such as pollen, and it lowers the humidity in the room or house. This reduces your risk of exposure to dust mites and your risk of having a flare-up. Exposure to cold weather may also cause a flare-up in some people.

Feathered and Furry Friends can Trigger Asthma

Pets and animals, while adorable, can trigger an asthma episode in people who are allergic to them. Dander is one trigger, and all animals have it (some more than others).

Additionally, proteins found in an animal's saliva, feces, urine, hair, and skin can trigger asthma. The best way to avoid a flare-up from these triggers is to avoid the animal altogether.

If you're not ready to part ways with a beloved family pet, try keeping the animal out of your bedroom, off furniture, and outside most of the time if possible. Indoor pets should be bathed frequently.

Be a Dust Detective

Dust mites, a common allergen, love to hide out in places and rooms we frequent, including bedrooms, living rooms, and offices. Purchase dust-proof covers for your mattress, box spring, and sofa. Buy dust-proof pillow wraps that go between your pillow and your pillowcase. Wash linens on the hottest water setting.

Carpets and rugs are dust magnets, too. If you have carpeting in your home, it may be time to bid adieu and have hardwood floors put down instead.

Don't be Friendly to Mold

Mold and mildew are two big asthma triggers. You can prevent flare-ups from these triggers by being aware of damp places in your kitchen, bath, basement, and around the yard. High humidity increases the risk for mold and mildew growth. Invest in a dehumidifier if humidity is a concern. Be sure to toss out any shower curtains, rugs, leaves, or firewood with mold or mildew.

Threats that Crawl

Cockroaches aren't just creepy; they can make you sick, too. These bugs and their droppings are a potential asthma trigger. If you discover a cockroach problem, take steps to eliminate them. Cover up, store, and remove open water and food containers. Vacuum, sweep, and mop any areas where you see cockroaches. Call an exterminator or use roach gels to reduce the number of bugs in your home. Don't forget to inspect your home's outside to see where bugs might be hiding.

4.2 Creating an Asthma Friendly Environment

Asthma care can involve a variety of treatments and approaches to managing your condition. Sometimes it is possible to make changes in the environment that help make life easier for you and/or people with asthma.

Make it a Smoke-free Zone: Be strict about smoking and vaping in your home. Sometimes people hesitate to insist that no smoking be allowed in their homes, but you might be surprised to learn that most people accept this kind of ban. In surveys, up to 90% of respondents report that their homes are smoke-free, including half of the smokers in one study. Air purifiers have been shown to have some effect on air quality in homes where people are allowed to smoke, but they are not as effective as stopping indoor smoking.

Clean Carefully: Frequent vacuuming, washing soft furnishings often, and dusting thoroughly can all help asthma sufferers. But you should also be cautious about the kinds of cleaning products you choose.

Feather dusters may send dust and dander into the air, triggering asthma attacks. Scented cleaners and spray cleaners can irritate the lungs. Try a liquid or gel cleaner instead, use unscented products, and open windows while you clean. In fact, it's best for people with asthma to let someone else do the cleaning. Swap chores to avoid contact with cleaners.

Neutralize Those Flowers: About 80% of people with asthma have allergies. Asthma triggers can include food allergies and sensitivity to dust or even insects. Allergies to flowers can be an issue since people bring flowers into homes and offices intentionally. Fortunately, removing the stamens of scented flowers like lilies removes the threat of an asthma attack. Just pinch off the anther (the pollen-containing part of the stamen) and dispose of it.

Avoid Scented Products: Air fresheners, essential oil diffusers, scented candles, incense, potpourri — many people enjoy these, but they can be torture for people with asthma. Keep your home well-ventilated unless outdoor air carries pollen or other allergens. In that case, wash your hands or even shower when you come inside, keep windows closed, and rely on air conditioning. Just be sure to keep ducts and filters clean.

Control Pets: Keep pets outside if possible. Bathe furry pets regularly and keep their spaces — crates or beds, for example — clean. Some pets are more likely to trigger allergies than others, and people's sensitivity varies, too. Poodles and other dogs of this type may be less likely to trigger an asthma attack than long-haired breeds. Parakeets may be less allergy-provoking than parrots. Apart from allergies, pet dander may cause breathing problems for people with asthma. If pets are important in your family, consider fish or turtles instead of furry friends.

4.3 Exercise, Nutrition and Asthma Control

Exercise and Asthma Control

Sometimes, aerobic exercise can trigger or worsen asthma-related symptoms. When this happens, it's called exercise-induced asthma or exercise-induced bronchoconstriction (EIB). You can have EIB even if you don't have asthma. If you do have EIB, you might be hesitant to workout. But having it doesn't mean you should avoid regular exercise. It's possible for people with EIB to workout with comfort and ease.

In fact, regular physical activity can decrease asthma symptoms by improving your lung health. The key is to do the right kind — and amount — of exercise. You can determine what this looks like for you by working with a doctor.

Can Exercise Stop Asthma Symptoms?

Some types of exercise can reduce or prevent asthma symptoms. They work by making your lungs stronger without worsening inflammation. Specifically, these activities minimize symptoms because they:

Increase endurance: Over time, working out can help your airways build up tolerance to exercise. This makes it easier for your lungs to perform activities that usually make you winded, like walking up stairs.

Reduce inflammation: Though asthma inflames the airways, regular exercise can actually decrease inflammation. It works by reducing inflammatory proteins, which improves how your airways respond to exercise.

Improve lung capacity: The more you work out, the more your lungs get used to consuming oxygen. This decreases how hard your body must work to breathe on a daily basis.

Strengthen muscle: When your muscles are strong, the body functions more efficiently during everyday activities.

Improve cardiovascular fitness: Exercise improves the overall conditioning of the heart, improving blood flow and the delivery of oxygen.

What Exercises are Best for People with Asthma?

In general, the best exercises for asthma involve brief bursts of exertion. Gentle, low-intensity activities are also ideal. These exercises don't overwork your lungs, so they're less likely to cause asthma symptoms. Everyone is different, though. Be sure to consult your doctor and pay attention to your body.

You can try:

Swimming: Swimming is one of the most recommended exercises for people with asthma. Compared to other activities, it's less likely to cause asthma-related symptoms due to:

- moist, warm air
- low pollen exposure
- pressure of fluid on the chest

Despite these benefits, chlorinated pools can cause symptoms in some individuals. Use caution if you're new to swimming in pools.

Walking: As a low-intensity activity, walking is another great choice. This form of exercise is gentle on the body, which makes it easier to breathe. For the most comfortable experience, only walk outside when it's warm. Dry, cool air can trigger or worsen your symptoms. You can also walk on a treadmill or indoor track.

Hiking: Another option is to enjoy a gentle hike. Choose a trail that's relatively flat or has a slow, steady incline. If you have allergies, check the local pollen count before hiking. Only hike if pollen levels are low.

Recreational Biking: If you have EIB, try biking at a leisurely pace. This is another gentle activity that doesn't involve constant exertion. You can also do indoor cycling on a stationary bike.

Short-distance Track and Field: If you'd like to run, opt for short-distance running activities such as sprints. Long-distance running on a track or outside may not be recommended in people with more uncontrolled asthma due to the ongoing effort required.

Nutrition and Asthma Control

If you have asthma, you may be curious about whether certain foods and diet choices could help you manage your condition. There's no conclusive evidence that a specific diet has an effect on the frequency or severity of asthma attacks.

At the same time, eating fresh, nutritious foods may improve your overall health as well as your asthma symptoms.

According to some research, a shift from eating fresh foods, such as fruits and vegetables, to processed foods may be linked to an increase in asthma cases in recent decades. Although more study is needed, early evidence suggests that there's no single food or nutrient that improves asthma symptoms on its own. Instead, people with asthma may benefit from eating a well-rounded diet high in fresh fruits and vegetables.

Food also comes into play as it relates to allergies. Food allergies and food intolerances occur when your immune system overreacts to specific proteins in foods. In some cases, this can result in asthma symptoms.

Foods to Add to your Diet
There's no specific diet recommended for asthma, but there are some foods and nutrients that may help support lung function:

Vitamin D: Getting enough vitamin D may help reduce the number of asthma attacks in children ages 6 to 15, according to the Vitamin D Council. Sources of vitamin D include:

- salmon

- milk and fortified milk

- fortified orange juice

- eggs

If you know you have allergies to milk or eggs, you may want to avoid them as a source of vitamin D. Allergic symptoms from a food source can manifest as asthma.

Vitamin A: A 2018 study found that children with asthma typically had lower levels of vitamin A in their blood than children without asthma. In children with asthma, higher levels of vitamin A also corresponded to better lung function. Good sources of vitamin A are:

- carrots

- cantaloupe

- sweet potatoes

- leafy greens, such as romaine lettuce, kale, and spinach
- broccoli

Apples: An apple a day may keep asthma away. According to a research review, apples were associated with a lower risk of asthma and increased lung function.

Bananas: According to research, bananas might decrease wheezing in children with asthma. This may be due to the fruit's antioxidant and potassium content, which may improve lung function.

Magnesium: A study found that children ages 11 to 19 who had low magnesium levels also had low lung flow and volume. Kids can improve their magnesium levels by eating magnesium-rich foods such as:

- spinach
- pumpkin seeds
- Swiss chard
- dark chocolate
- salmon

Inhaling magnesium through a nebulizer) is another good way to treat asthma attacks.

Foods to Avoid

Some foods may trigger asthma symptoms and should be avoided. However, it's best to consult your doctor before you start eliminating certain foods from your diet.

Sulfites: Sulfites are a type of preservative that may worsen asthma. They're found in:

- wine

- dried fruits

- pickled food

- maraschino cherries

- shrimp

- bottled lemon and lime juice

Foods that Cause Gas: Eating large meals or foods that cause gas will put pressure on your diaphragm, especially if you have acid reflux. This may cause chest tightness and trigger asthma flares. These foods include:

- beans

- cabbage

- carbonated drinks

- onions

- garlic

- fried foods

Salicylates: Although it's rare, some people with asthma may be sensitive to salicylates found in coffee, tea, and some herbs and spices. Salicylates are naturally occurring chemical compounds, and they're sometimes found in foods.

Artificial Ingredients: Chemical preservatives, flavorings, and colorings are often found in processed and fast food. Some people with asthma may be sensitive or allergic to these artificial ingredients.

Chapter 5: Treatment Options and Medication

5.1 Inhalers: Types and Usage

An inhaler is a small, handheld device that delivers medication directly to your lungs. Inhalers can be dry powder, metered-dose or soft mist. The most common types use medicine that helps open your airways or reduce inflammation in your lungs.

What are the Different Types of Inhalers?

Types of inhaler devices include pressurized metered dose inhalers (pMDIs), dry powder inhalers (DPIs) and soft mist inhalers.

Metered Dose Inhalers: Metered dose inhalers (MDIs or pMDIs), sometimes called "puffers," hold the medication in a pressurized canister. The canister sits in a handheld container with a mouthpiece. When you press on the canister, a propellant (something that helps the medicine move out of the canister) helps send a puff of medicine out of the mouthpiece. Following the directions, you breathe the puff in through your mouth to pull the medicine into your lungs. MDIs deliver one dose at a time from a canister that holds multiple doses.

Dry Powder Inhalers: Dry powder inhalers (DPIs) store medicine as a powder inside capsules or other containers that you activate when you're ready to use the inhaler. Unlike MDIs, a propellant doesn't push the medicine out of a DPI. Instead, you use a quick, deep breath to pull the powder out and into your lungs.

DPIs are usually tube- or disk-shaped, with a mouthpiece. Some have a place to load medicine. Different styles and brands have different instructions on how to activate and use them. Some examples of dry powder inhaler devices include:

- Twisthaler
- Flexhaler
- Diskus
- HandiHaler
- Ellipta
- Breezhaler

Soft Mist Inhalers: Soft mist inhalers (Respimat) turn liquid medicine into a fine mist. You breathe the mist in through your mouth to get the medicine to your lungs.

How Do You Use an Inhaler?

Each inhaler device has its own directions. Make sure you follow the directions for your specific device and ask your provider to show you how to use it. General directions include:

- Open or take the cap off the inhaler.
- For metered-dose inhalers, you may need to prime your inhaler by shaking it and spraying it into the air as directed. For some dry powder inhalers, such as Diskus, you may need to load a dose as directed.
- Breathe out as much air as you possibly can from your lungs.
- Put the inhaler in your mouth.
- With a metered-dose inhaler, you'll need to breathe in slowly through your mouth and press down on the canister. This timing is different depending on whether you're using a spacer (a tube attached to

the end of the mouthpiece). With a dry powder inhaler, you breathe in quickly and deeply. Your breath pulls the medicine out of the inhaler. With a soft mist inhaler, you'll release a dose while breathing in slowly.

- Hold your breath for 10 seconds to allow the medicine to reach your lungs.
- Rinse out your mouth and spit after using an ICS inhaler to prevent thrush.

5.2 Long-Term Controllers vs Quick-Relief

Long-term controllers Also called "maintenance" or "long-term preventative" inhalers, controller inhalers are taken every day on a long-term basis to improve control of asthma, improve asthma symptoms, and help prevent asthma attacks. Controller inhalers are inhaled corticosteroid medications that reduce and prevent asthmatic inflammation in the lungs. (The inhaled corticosteroids used to treat asthma are not the same as the steroids that some athletes take illegally. Inhaled corticosteroids for asthma are used at a low dose and rarely cause any side effects.) Because controller inhalers take a few days to start working, you will not feel any benefit from taking controller inhalers right away – so, it is very important to take these medications regularly, even if your asthma is under control (and don't stop controller inhalers during an asthma flare!). Controller inhalers taken every day are the primary asthma treatment for all but the mildest types of asthma

On the other hand, quick-relief medications are short-acting medications (such as albuterol or levalbuterol) that temporarily relieve wheezing and shortness of breath. They might help stop a mild asthma flare, but quick-relief inhalers do not prevent serious asthma attacks, and they do not provide long-term protection; if you are taking multiple puffs of a quick-relief inhaler in a single day, you need to see your physician to change your asthma medications. For some types of asthma, quick-relief inhalers can also be used before exercise; talk to your doctor before attempting this.

5.3   Alternative   Therapies   and Complementary Treatments

In recent years, there has been a growing interest in alternative therapies and complementary treatments as individuals seek holistic approaches to health and well-being. These practices, often used in conjunction with conventional medicine, aim to address the physical, mental, and emotional aspects of an individual's health. Let's look at the concept of alternative therapies and the role they play in enhancing overall wellness.

First, alternative therapies encompass a broad range of non-conventional healing practices that fall outside the realm of mainstream medicine. These may include acupuncture, chiropractic care, herbal medicine, homeopathy, and more. Unlike conventional medicine, alternative therapies often emphasize a holistic approach, considering the interconnectedness of the body, mind, and spirit. They aim to restore balance and promote self-healing.

Complementary treatments are used alongside traditional medical approaches to enhance the overall effectiveness of the treatment plan. In many cases, they sought to alleviate the side effects of conventional medical interventions, such as pain, nausea, or emotional distress.

Common Types of Alternative Therapies and Complementary Treatments
Acupuncture and Acupressure: Based on traditional Chinese medicine, these therapies involve stimulating specific points on the body to promote energy flow and balance.

Herbal Medicine: The use of plants and plant extracts for their therapeutic properties, addressing various health concerns.

Mind-Body Practices: Meditation, yoga, and tai chi are examples that focus on the connection between mental and physical well-being.

Massage Therapy: Manipulation of soft tissues to promote relaxation, reduce stress, and alleviate physical discomfort.

It's crucial for individuals to communicate openly with their healthcare providers about any alternative or complementary treatments they are considering. While many alternative therapies offer benefits, not all have undergone rigorous scientific testing. Understanding the potential risks and benefits is essential.

Chapter 6: Asthma in Different Life Stages

6.1 Managing Childhood Asthma

For most kids with asthma, their symptoms can be controlled — sometimes so well that flare-ups are rare. But learning about asthma (what treatments to take and when, what triggers to avoid and when) can be the hardest part of asthma care.

Don't be discouraged. Learn as much as you can, talk to others living with asthma, read up on asthma, and discuss any concerns with your child's doctor. Once you and your family are used to dealing with asthma, it will become a normal part of your routine. These tips can help:

Have a Plan and Stick to It: Your child should have an asthma action plan. These written instructions from the doctor give clear, step-by-step directions on what medicines to take and when, how to avoid triggers, what to do between flare-ups, and how to recognize and manage them if they happen. By following this plan, you will learn how to care for your child and when to call the doctor for help.

Take Medicines as Prescribed: Most kids with asthma need to take medicines. Some are daily medicines that work over time to ease or prevent inflamed (irritated and swollen) airways. Others are used only during a flare-up to help open the airways. Some can do both things at the same time. Most medicines call for the use of a nebulizer or inhaler with a spacer to help get medicine into the lungs. Sometimes medicine is given as a pill or liquid. The doctor will tell you which medicines your child needs and how to take them.

Identify and Avoid Triggers: Triggers are things that can bother airways and lead to an asthma flare-up. Common triggers are allergens like pollen and mold, weather changes, and viral infections (like the common cold). Finding your child's triggers can take some work, but it's worth it. The doctor can help too — for instance, testing your child for allergies if you think they're making the asthma worse. When you know the triggers, help your child avoid them as much as possible.

Know the Signs of a Flare-up: After your child has had a few flare-ups, you may start to notice when one is going to happen. Early warning signs can help you spot a flare-up hours or even a day before obvious symptoms (such as wheezing and coughing) start. Kids can have changes in how they look, their mood or breathing, or they'll complain of "feeling funny" in some way. Be sure you know your child's signs and are ready to adjust medicines or give them, as needed.

Know What to do for a Severe Flare-up: Know when your child's symptoms call for medical care, or even a trip to the emergency room (ER). Always have asthma medicine available for the quick relief of symptoms in case your child needs it — everyone who cares for your child (like teachers and coaches) also should know when and how to give the medicine.

6.2 Asthma in Adolescents and Young Adults

Millions of adolescents suffer from asthma all over the world. As it is one of the most common and well-known respiratory conditions, it is understandable that young adults and adolescents face several challenges because of it. These challenges often result in the disruption of daily life and activities. As a result, being able to manage asthma and having coping techniques to face such obstacles is critical.

The following are some of the most typical obstacles that teenagers with asthma confront, as well as their associated coping strategies:

Stigma: An aspect that many fail to consider about asthma in young adults and adolescents is the stigma that they often feel or experience. Some adolescents with asthma may feel stigmatized by their condition, particularly if they need to use inhalers or avoid certain activities. Young adolescents frequently lose confidence because of feeling left out or being unable to participate in strenuous activities. As a result of their condition, some young people may be shunned by their peers.

Coping strategy: To eliminate stigma and promote understanding, the greatest coping method for such a situation is to educate classmates and teachers about asthma. Furthermore, encouraging teenagers with asthma to have a more positive self-image despite their condition will help them overcome any stigma they may feel.

Medication adherence: Adhering to prescribed medication is a must when it comes to addressing asthma. Adolescents may forget to take their asthma medication or resist taking it due to side effects. This can result in the aggravation of their condition, causing greater discomfort and difficulty in breathing.

Coping strategy: One of the most effective ways to overcome this challenge is to develop a routine for taking medication. Involving affected kids in the formulation and maintenance of their own treatment plan can also help establish a good and attentive attitude toward medication adherence. Using respiratory aids like portable nebulizers help in maintaining adherence to medication.

Exercise Limitations: Often, exercise can prompt asthma to kick in which can cause additional discomfort and discourage affected teenagers and adolescents from any form of manual work. Exercise-induced asthma can limit adolescents' ability to participate in sports or other physical activities which can adversely affect their overall performance in life.

Coping strategy: Working with healthcare providers to develop an asthma action plan that includes medication before exercise, warm-up, and cool-down can help prevent any exercise induced asthma attacks. This enables for the continuation of light physical activity and exercise, which can aid in healthier breathing.

Peer Pressure: As impressionable individuals, adolescents with asthma may feel peer pressure to smoke or vape. A want to connect with others of the same and a pressure to be accepted and be "normal" by others can also cause adolescents with asthma to pick up harmful habits early which will only aggravate their condition.

Coping strategy: Educate adolescents about the risks of smoking and vaping and encourage healthy behaviors.

Emotional Distress: Being unable to breathe might naturally induce emotional anguish. Adolescents with asthma may experience anxiety or depression related to their condition. When suffering an asthma episode, teenagers frequently panic.

Coping Strategy: The best coping strategy for such cases is to seek professional support. Getting help from a professional like therapists and nurses can help adolescents overcome their anxiety and depression, while also teaching them to remain calm and composed when panicking.

School Attendance: Asthma symptoms may cause mental block or fatigue which can be seen to affect teenagers' desire to attend school. Adolescents can be more prone to miss school or struggle academically when suffering from inhibiting conditions like asthma and COPD. Asthmatic children are more likely to drop out of school before the age of 16 and to drop out of college or university.

Coping strategy: Creating a plan alongside the teachers and school staff for the addressing and management of asthma symptoms can help establish confidence and security in the minds of young children, leading to the minimization of disruption to academic performance.

By addressing these challenges and developing coping strategies, adolescents with asthma can improve their quality of life and manage their condition effectively. A multidisciplinary approach that includes healthcare providers, educators, and mental health providers can be effective in supporting adolescents with asthma.

6.3 Asthma in the Elderly

Late-onset asthma can be challenging to diagnose in the elderly due to several reasons. Older adults often suffer from other health issues, which may result in the misdiagnosis of asthma. Lung function tests may pose problems, and medicines used for other conditions can further complicate the diagnosis. Additionally, age-related illnesses such as chronic obstructive pulmonary disease (COPD), congestive heart failure, acid reflux disease (GERD), and paroxysmal arrhythmias make it more difficult to diagnose asthma in older adults. Certain medications such as heart medicines, cholinergic agents, aspirin, and non-steroidal anti-inflammatories (NSAIDs) can tighten airways and exacerbate asthma symptoms. If you suspect that your elderly loved one has onset asthma, it is vital to take them to a doctor who can perform physical exams and lung function tests and review their medical and family history.

Treatment of asthma in the elderly is vital if your loved one has been diagnosed. When it comes to controlling asthma in seniors, it is important to explore all available treatment options beyond inhalers. Below are some tips for managing asthma in seniors, as well as alternative treatment options to consider.

Reduce or Avoid Triggers: This can include cold air, weather changes, smoke, pollution, or even strong emotions.

Take Prescribed Medications: These can work to relieve symptoms after asthma symptoms flare up or even prevent inflammation in your airways. This may include an asthma inhaler for elderly individuals.

Talk to a Physician: Speak to a professional about a proper action plan. This can include taking note of when symptoms get worse and taking note of what to do in an extreme emergency.

Monitor Overall Health: Asthma shouldn't necessarily be treated on its own. Other medical conditions or illnesses, such as allergies, can make asthma worse. Be sure to keep all of these other conditions in check.

Chapter 7: Living Well with Asthma

7.1 Coping Strategies and Emotional Support

Living with asthma necessitates a holistic approach that extends beyond managing physical symptoms. Effective coping strategies empower individuals to navigate the challenges associated with this chronic condition, fostering resilience and improving overall well-being.

Education and Self-awareness: Understanding asthma is foundational to effective coping. Education empowers individuals to identify triggers, comprehend medications, and adopt proactive self-management techniques. By gaining insights into their condition, individuals develop a sense of control, reducing anxiety associated with unpredictability.

Breathing Techniques: Practicing specific breathing exercises serves as a powerful tool for stress reduction and symptom management during asthma attacks. Techniques like diaphragmatic breathing and pursed lip breathing promote relaxation, aiding individuals in regaining control over their respiratory function.

Physical Activity: Engaging in regular, moderate physical activity contributes to overall well-being and respiratory health. Exercise strengthens respiratory muscles, improves lung function, and boosts immunity. Individuals can work with healthcare professionals to tailor exercise plans that align with their capabilities and preferences.

Journaling: Keeping a journal to track symptoms, triggers, and emotional states provides valuable insights for effective asthma management. This practice helps individuals identify patterns, recognize potential triggers, and communicate more effectively with healthcare providers. Journaling serves as a personal tool for self-reflection and empowerment.

These coping strategies empower individuals to actively participate in their asthma management, fostering a proactive and resilient mindset.

When it comes to emotional support, it's important to remember that there is no one-size-fits-all solution. What works for one person may not work for another. Let's look at ways you can get emotional support.

Building a Supportive Network: Open communication with family and friends establishes a crucial support system. Educating close contacts about asthma symptoms, medications, and potential emergencies creates a supportive environment. Sharing experiences and challenges with loved ones fosters understanding and empathy.

Support Groups: Participation in asthma support groups, whether in-person or online, provides individuals with a sense of community. Peer support offers empathy, encouragement, and practical advice for coping with the emotional aspects of asthma. Shared experiences create a supportive environment where individuals feel understood and validated.

Professional Support: Seeking guidance from mental health professionals, such as psychologists or counselors, can be instrumental in addressing emotional challenges associated with chronic conditions like asthma. Professionals can provide coping strategies, stress management techniques, and a safe space for individuals to express their concerns and fears.

Incorporating Mind-Body Practices: Mindfulness and meditation practices offer valuable tools for stress reduction. Incorporating these techniques into daily routines promotes emotional well-being and helps individuals manage anxiety related to their condition.

Additionally, yoga, which combines physical activity, controlled breathing, and mindfulness, has shown positive effects in improving asthma symptoms and emotional resilience.

Effective Communication with Healthcare Providers: Establishing open and transparent communication with healthcare providers is crucial for emotional support. Discussing emotional concerns, treatment preferences, and fears fosters a collaborative approach to asthma management. Shared decision-making ensures that individuals feel heard and actively participate in their care plan.

Crisis Preparedness: Developing and understanding emergency action plans empowers individuals to respond effectively to worsening symptoms. Knowing when and how to seek medical assistance reduces anxiety and promotes a sense of preparedness. Having a well-defined plan in place provides a tangible strategy for managing crisis situations.

Routine Monitoring and Self-Care: Consistent follow-up with healthcare providers ensures ongoing asthma management. Regular check-ups address both physical and emotional aspects of the condition. Prioritizing self-care practices, including adequate sleep, a balanced diet, and stress management, contributes to overall resilience and improved asthma outcomes.

7.2 Overcoming Stigma with Misconceptions

Living with a medical condition often comes with not only physical challenges but also the weight of societal attitudes and misconceptions. Overcoming stigma is a crucial aspect of the journey for individuals dealing with various health issues, including asthma. Here's a guide on navigating and overcoming stigma and misconceptions associated with asthma:

Understanding the Stigma: Stigma surrounding asthma often stems from misunderstandings about the condition. Asthma is sometimes perceived as a minor inconvenience rather than a chronic respiratory condition that can significantly impact daily life. This misunderstanding may lead to societal misconceptions, including the belief that individuals with asthma are not as capable or healthy as their peers.

Educating Others: One of the most effective ways to combat stigma is through education. Individuals with asthma can play a pivotal role in dispelling misconceptions by sharing accurate information about the condition. This may involve explaining that asthma is a chronic condition characterized by inflammation of the airways, and it requires ongoing management rather than being a temporary inconvenience.

Open Communication: Creating an open dialogue about asthma helps break down barriers and fosters understanding. Individuals can share their experiences, challenges, and triumphs, providing insight into the realities of living with asthma. Open communication helps humanize the condition and dispels myths that may contribute to stigmatization.

Challenging Stereotypes: Stereotypes about asthma may include assumptions about physical capabilities, work performance, or lifestyle choices. Individuals with asthma can challenge these stereotypes by actively participating in various activities, showcasing that asthma does not define one's abilities. This can be particularly powerful in workplace settings, where proving competence can contribute to changing perceptions.

Advocacy and Awareness Campaigns: Engaging in advocacy and awareness campaigns on asthma helps bring the condition into the spotlight. By participating in or supporting initiatives that aim to educate the public, individuals with asthma contribute to breaking down stigmas. These campaigns can focus on dispelling myths, sharing personal stories, and promoting a broader understanding of the challenges faced by those with asthma.

Seeking Professional Support: Sometimes, the impact of stigma and misconceptions on mental well-being requires professional support. Mental health professionals can assist individuals in developing coping strategies, building resilience, and addressing the emotional toll that societal attitudes may take.

Empowering Self-Advocacy: Empowering individuals with asthma to become advocates for themselves is a key strategy. This involves providing them with the tools and confidence to communicate their needs, rights, and capabilities. Self-advocacy not only contributes to personal empowerment but also fosters a culture of respect and understanding.

Building a Support Network: Creating a strong support network is essential in overcoming stigma. Family, friends, colleagues, and fellow individuals with asthma can offer understanding, encouragement, and solidarity. Knowing that one is not alone in the journey can be empowering and helps counteract the isolating effects of stigma.

Chapter 8: Asthma Management in Specific Situations

8.1 Asthma and Pregnancy

If you're pregnant or are thinking about becoming pregnant, it's more important than ever to keep your asthma controlled. Avoiding triggers and taking your asthma medications as prescribed can all help ensure a healthy pregnancy for you and your baby-to-be.

A national expert panel strongly encourages monthly monitoring of asthma during prenatal visits. This is because the course of asthma improves for about one-third of women and worsens for about one-third of women during pregnancy. A monthly evaluation gives your physician the opportunity to step down treatment (if possible) or increase treatment (if necessary). Asthma attacks are most common during the later weeks of pregnancy, but are very rare during labor itself.

Managing Your Asthma During Pregnancy
Good asthma control is crucial for a healthy pregnancy. An asthma flare-up causes decreased oxygen levels in the blood. This, in turn, can lead to less oxygen reaching the fetus. Low oxygen can impair healthy fetal growth and development.

To minimize risk, pregnant women should avoid allergens that trigger their symptoms. Also, women who smoke should quit prior to getting pregnant as smoking may trigger asthma and can interfere with fetal development.

If you were receiving allergy shots (immunotherapy) prior to becoming pregnant, you can continue this treatment during pregnancy. Just be sure to let your doctor know that you are pregnant. It is not recommended to start allergy shots during pregnancy.

What About Medications?

Continue to see your allergist/immunologist throughout your pregnancy and don't stop taking your medications. Many mothers-to-be are concerned about taking medications during pregnancy. Yet the risks posed by uncontrolled asthma are much greater than those from asthma treatments.

Inhaled corticosteroids are often the treatment of choice for persistent asthma. Studies have shown them to be effective and low-risk for pregnant women. The National Asthma Education and Prevention Program (NAEPP) recommends two specific drugs: budesonide (inhaled corticosteroid) and albuterol (short-acting Beta 2-agonist) as having good safety profiles when used during pregnancy.

Oral corticosteroids are not preferred for regular asthma treatment during pregnancy. However they can be used to treat severe asthma attacks.

If you are pregnant and think you may have asthma, it's important to have your condition diagnosed to reduce the risks to your baby. Studies have linked asthma attacks in early pregnancy to birth defects, so don't wait to have your condition diagnosed.

8.2 Occupational Asthma

Approximately 10 to 25 percent of adults with asthma experience occupational asthma. Occupational asthma is a type of asthma caused by exposure to inhaled irritants in the workplace. It is often a reversible condition, which means the symptoms may disappear when the irritants that caused the asthma are avoided. However, permanent damage can result if the person experiences prolonged exposure. Examples of workplace irritants include:

- Dusts
- Gasses
- Fumes
- Vapors

Occupational asthma symptoms are the same as any asthma exacerbation, such as wheezing, shortness of breath, runny nose, nasal congestion, eye irritation, and chest tightness. These symptoms may get worse during exposure to the irritant(s) at work. The cause can be allergic or non allergic in nature. Symptoms may get better when the person is not at work. Sometimes, occupational asthma symptoms do not appear until several hours after the exposure, even while at home after work. At the onset of the disease, symptoms may subside during weekends and vacations, but exposure to an occupational irritant can cause asthma within 24 hours. However, during later stages of occupational asthma, asthma symptoms may become a problem during exposure to other, more common asthma triggers, such as smoke, dust, and temperature changes.

How can Occupational Asthma be Managed/Prevented?

Avoidance of triggers is the best prevention against asthma. If occupational asthma symptoms do occur, you may need to change jobs to avoid exposure. However, certain steps taken in the workplace can help reduce the risk of occupational asthma:

- Change the work process to better handle irritant exposure

- Use industrial hygiene techniques that are appropriate for the type of irritant you are exposed to and that will keep exposure levels to a minimum

- Have regular medical checkups to identify possible damage that may be occurring to the lungs or other medical conditions specifically related to the irritant exposure

- Be aware of any personal and/or family medical history of asthma which may put you at greater risk for occupational asthma in certain industries

8.3 Traveling with Asthma: Tips and Precautions

Actively avoiding your triggers can reduce your risk of an asthma attack. But when you're traveling, it's hard to know what triggers might pop up during your trip.

Because new environments can be unpredictable, it's important to be prepared. Enjoy your vacation — while avoiding an allergic asthma attack — by taking these simple steps.

Stay on Top of Your Treatment Plan: Allergic asthma can usually be managed with daily medications and rescue inhalers. If you're still having symptoms even though you follow your treatment plan, you may need to reevaluate it with your doctor. The best way to stay healthy on your trip is to be as healthy and well-prepared as possible before you go.

Be Strategic When Planning Your Travel: Consider if you're more likely to encounter certain triggers if you journey to certain places. You may want to choose your destination with your triggers in mind. If your symptoms are triggered by mold spores, avoid vacationing in damp, rainy regions and stay away from older, potentially musty buildings.

If your symptoms are triggered by air pollution, don't go to major urban areas where air quality is generally lower. You may also want to avoid regions with high pollen counts in the spring and fall.

Being strategic about your destination can boost your health and happiness during your trip.

See Your Doctor: Before you leave, schedule a check-up with your doctor. They'll be able to refill prescriptions and review travel-related risks. They can also give you any immunizations you need, like the flu shot. Your doctor should also provide a letter explaining your condition, and include medications or devices you may need in case of a medical emergency.

If you haven't yet, work with your doctor to develop an allergic asthma action plan. It should include what to do in case of an emergency, a list of your prescription medications, and your doctor's name and contact information.

Check Allergy Policies: If you're traveling by plane, train, or bus, check out the travel company's allergy policies. Ask questions like:

- Are animals permitted onboard? If so, may I be seated several rows away?
- Are allergy-safe meals provided? If not, may I bring my own food?
- May I pre-board to wipe down my seating area?
- Is smoking allowed? Is there a non-smoking section available to book?

Dedicating a few minutes to researching allergy policies can make all the difference when it comes to having a safe, comfortable trip.

Pack Your Medication in Your Carry-on: It's vital to keep your allergic asthma medications and devices with you at all times. That means packing your supplies in your carry-on luggage and keeping them on-hand for the entirety of your trip.
Checked luggage can be lost, damaged, or stolen. Depending on your destination, it may be hard to find the right replacement medications.

Don't Forget Your Devices: Be sure to pack any asthma devices that you use, such as a spacer or peak flow meter. If you use an electric nebulizer to manage allergic asthma, find out if you need an adapter for foreign electrical outlets. All of your devices should be packed in your carry-on luggage, too.

Book a Non-Smoking, Pet-Free Hotel Room: When booking your accommodations, be sure to request a non-smoking, pet-free room. This will help you avoid tobacco residue and pet dander. If your hotel can't guarantee a smoke-free and pet-free room, consider staying elsewhere.

Know the Nearest Hospital and the Local Emergency Number: Find the closest hospital to where you'll be staying. Figure out how you'll get to the hospital in an emergency. Different countries use different numbers to call for an ambulance. Here are some examples of national emergency numbers:
- in the United States and Canada, call 911
- in the European Union, call 112

- in the United Kingdom, call 999 or 112

- in Australia, call 000

- in New Zealand, call 111

Not all countries have well-developed emergency response systems. Find out the best way for you to get help quickly if you need it.

Know Asthma First-Aid: Learning how to care for yourself during an asthma attack could save your life. Remember these basic steps if you're having an asthma attack:

- Use your rescue medication right away.

- If your medication doesn't seem to be working, seek emergency medical help.

- Let someone know what's happening and ask them to stay with you.

- Stay in an upright position. *Don't lie down.

- Try to stay calm, since panicking may worsen symptoms.

- Try to take slow, steady breaths.

If symptoms persist or worsen, continue to take your rescue medication following your doctor's directions for use in an emergency, while you wait for medical help.

Don't hesitate to seek emergency medical help for asthma symptoms. Asthma attacks can worsen suddenly and unexpectedly.

Chapter 9: Building a Support Network

9.1 The Role of Family and Friends

Living with asthma is not a solitary journey; it is a shared experience that profoundly influences not only the individual with the condition but also those closest to them—family and friends. The role of this support network is invaluable, contributing significantly to the overall well-being and effective management of asthma. Here's a closer look at the indispensable role that family and friends play in navigating the challenges of asthma:

Emotional Support: Living with a chronic condition like asthma can be emotionally taxing. Family and friends serve as pillars of emotional support, providing comfort, understanding, and empathy during difficult times. The reassurance of knowing that loved ones are there for both the good and challenging moments can alleviate stress and anxiety.

Practical Assistance: Asthma management often involves practical considerations, from ensuring a home environment that minimizes triggers to helping with daily tasks during asthma flares. Family and friends can play a hands-on role in supporting the individual with asthma by assisting with chores, creating an asthma-friendly living space, or providing transportation during healthcare visits.

Medication Reminders: Consistent adherence to medication is critical for effective asthma management. Family and friends can play a pivotal role in reminding the individual to take their prescribed medications, ensuring that the treatment plan is followed diligently. This support is particularly vital during busy or stressful periods when medication routines might be disrupted.

Emergency Preparedness: Asthma emergencies, though rare, require prompt and appropriate action. Family and friends can be educated on the signs of an impending asthma attack and the necessary steps to take during an emergency. This knowledge equips them to respond effectively and seek medical assistance when needed.

Creating a Supportive Environment: Asthma triggers can vary, and creating a supportive environment is crucial. Family and friends can contribute by being mindful of potential triggers, such as smoke or allergens, and taking steps to minimize exposure. This collaborative effort fosters an environment that promotes respiratory health and well-being.

Encouragement for Physical Activity: Regular exercise is beneficial for individuals with asthma, and family and friends can encourage and engage in physical activities together. Whether it's a walk in the park or participation in asthma-friendly sports, the support of loved ones promotes a healthy and active lifestyle.

Advocacy in Social Settings: In social situations, friends and family can serve as advocates, helping educate others about asthma and dispelling misconceptions. Their understanding and proactive advocacy contribute to creating inclusive environments where the individual with asthma feels supported and accepted.

Monitoring and Communication: Family and friends are often in a unique position to notice changes in the individual's asthma symptoms. Open communication allows for the sharing of concerns and facilitates proactive management. Regular check-ins on well-being and discussions about asthma management strategies enhance the overall support system.

9.2   Joining   Support   Groups   and Communities

Living with asthma can be a unique journey, but the challenges and triumphs become more manageable when shared within a supportive community. Joining asthma-specific support groups and communities provides individuals with a wealth of benefits, ranging from emotional support to practical insights on managing the condition. Here's a closer look at the impact of being part of these communities:

Emotional Support: Asthma can be emotionally challenging, and connecting with others who share similar experiences creates a sense of understanding and camaraderie. Support groups offer a safe space for individuals to express their feelings, fears, and successes, fostering a sense of belonging and reducing the sense of isolation that sometimes accompanies chronic conditions.

Shared Experiences and Insights: Within these communities, individuals can exchange practical insights on managing asthma effectively. From tips on recognizing triggers to advice on adhering to medication regimens, the collective wisdom of the group becomes a valuable resource. Learning from the experiences of others can empower individuals to better navigate their own asthma journey.

Education and Awareness: Support groups often provide a platform for educational initiatives and awareness campaigns. Members can stay updated on the latest research, treatment options, and lifestyle strategies for asthma management. This continuous learning not only empowers individuals but also contributes to a more informed and proactive community.

Coping Strategies and Resilience: Sharing coping strategies for dealing with the challenges of asthma is a significant benefit of being part of a community. Members can discuss how they handle flare-ups, cope with stress, and maintain a positive mindset. This exchange of strategies fosters resilience and equips individuals with a toolbox of approaches to navigate various aspects of their asthma journey.

Advocacy and Empowerment: Collective advocacy is a potent force in raising awareness about asthma and advocating for better policies and resources. Support groups often engage in advocacy initiatives, promoting a broader understanding of asthma within society. Through these efforts, individuals find empowerment not only within the community but also in contributing to broader societal changes.

Practical Tips for Daily Living: Practical aspects of daily living with asthma, such as creating asthma-friendly environments at home and work, are frequent topics of discussion in support groups. Members share tips and hacks that make daily life more comfortable and less stressful. This practical knowledge can significantly enhance the quality of life for individuals with asthma.

Building Lasting Connections: Joining a support group can lead to the formation of lasting connections and friendships. The shared bond of living with asthma creates a unique camaraderie, and members often find comfort and encouragement in knowing they are not alone. These connections extend beyond the virtual or physical meeting spaces, providing ongoing support.

Conclusion: Embracing a Life with Asthma

Living with asthma can be challenging, but with the right treatment and support, it is possible to live a full and active life. In conclusion, here are some key takeaways:

- Acknowledge your emotions and seek support from friends, family, and healthcare professionals.
- Create an asthma action plan with your doctor and follow it closely.
- Avoid triggers, such as allergens and smoke.
- Stay active and make healthy lifestyle choices.

- Embrace life with asthma by finding things you enjoy doing, despite your condition.

Remember, you are not alone in your journey with asthma. Many people have learned to manage their asthma and live full and active lives. One example is Olympic swimmer, Amy Van Dyken. Van Dyken was diagnosed with asthma as a child, but she didn't let it hold her back. She went on to become one of the most decorated swimmers in U.S. history, winning six Olympic gold medals and a bronze medal. Van Dyken has said that her asthma has actually made her a better athlete, as it has taught her the importance of breathing control and proper technique.

This is just one example of how people with asthma can achieve their goals and lead fulfilling lives. Everyone's journey is unique, and there's no "one-size-fits-all" approach to living with asthma. Some people may need more medical intervention than others, and some may need to make more significant lifestyle changes. But everyone has the power to make choices that can positively impact their health.

If you're reading this book, Breathing Easy, you may also be interested in my books on Cystic fibrosis and Lung Cancer. Tap the links to read them.

Thank you for purchasing my book. I'd really appreciate it if you could take a moment to leave a review. Your feedback will help me improve and make my next book even better. I'm always looking forward to improving, so please do not hold back! Thank you for your time and support.